When Someone You Know Has Cancer™

Recommended for Young Adult Readers

Written by: Jean Schoen

Illustrated by: Greg Justus

DEDICATION

I dedicate this book to my three beautiful daughters whose lives were impacted by our experience and mistakes. Thank you for believing in me and in my mission, despite the rough times. I love you forever.

What Is Cancer?

Our bodies are made up of many different parts that all work together.

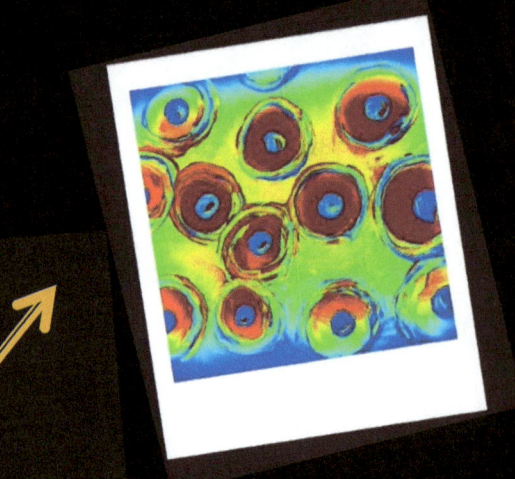

The smallest part is called a cell, and is so small that it can only be seen under a microscope.

The cells are the building blocks of the body.

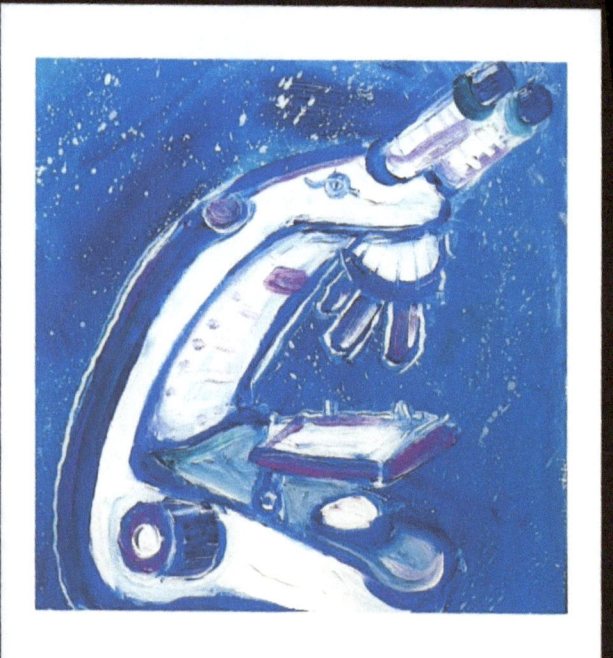

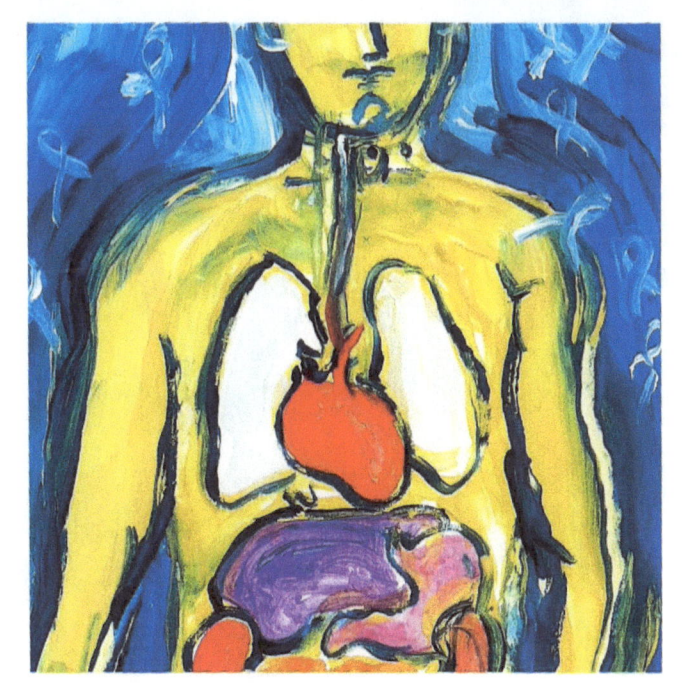

Large groups of cells are called tissues, and tissues that work together are called organs.

Organs, like our heart and lungs, allow us to live and fight against illness.

Sometimes changes occur to some of the cells, and these "sick" cells group together. When they do, it can damage organs and make a person very ill.

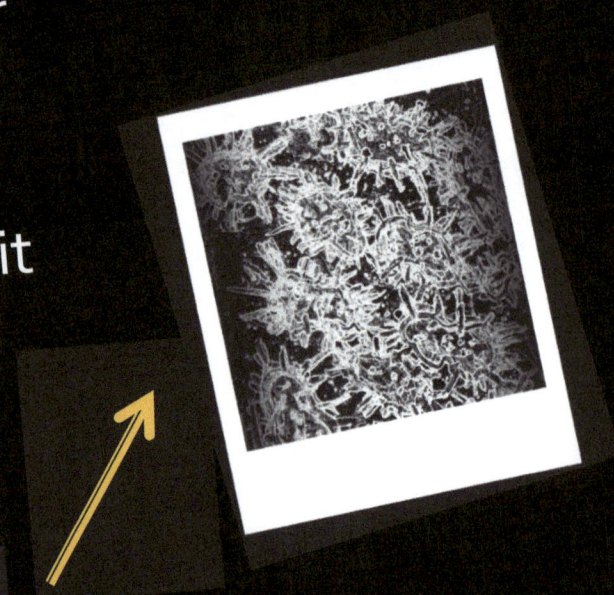

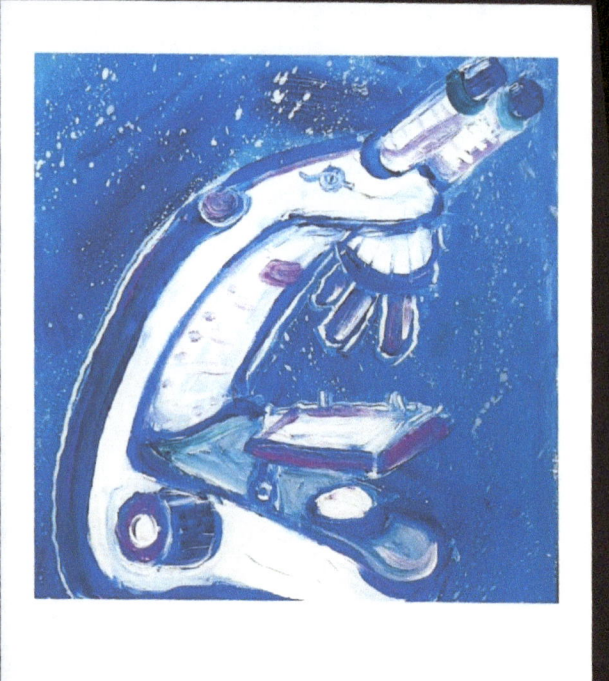

This is called **cancer**.

Cancer can happen to someone at any age, at any time.

Cancer can be very scary...
but it also can be treatable.

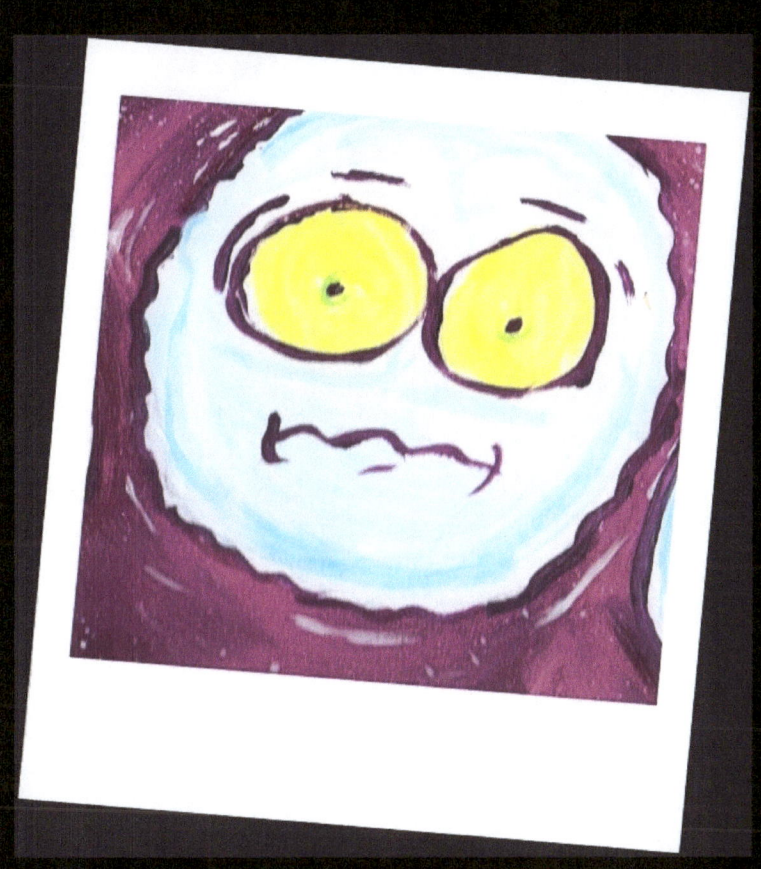

Cancer Treatments

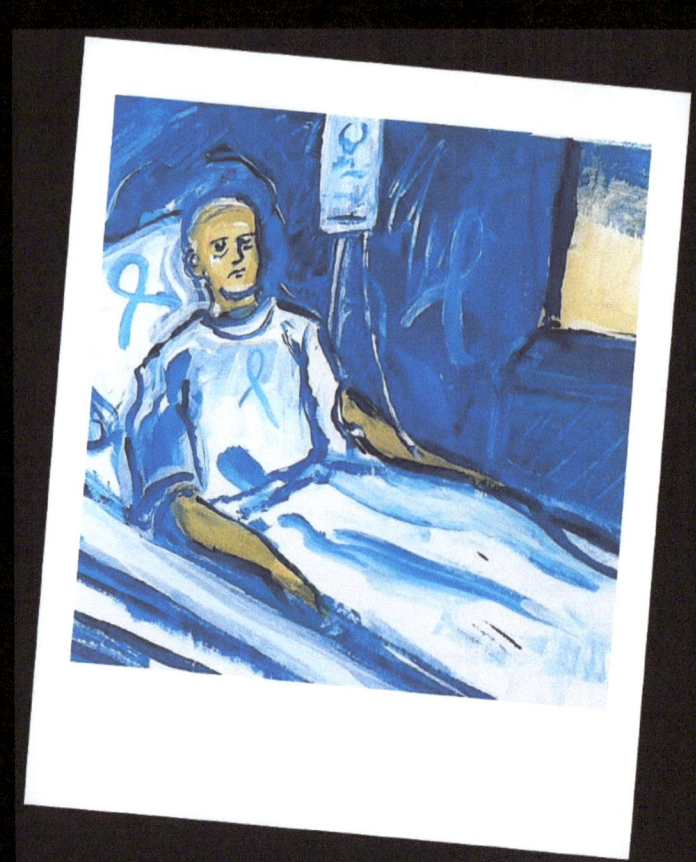

Doctors use medicines called **chemotherapy** to treat cancer. Chemotherapy kills the cancer cells but, unfortunately, also kills the healthy cells.

When a person receives chemo, a lot of different side effects can occur.

Some of the possible side effects are an upset stomach and decreased appetite. Another side effect you may notice is that their hair could fall out.

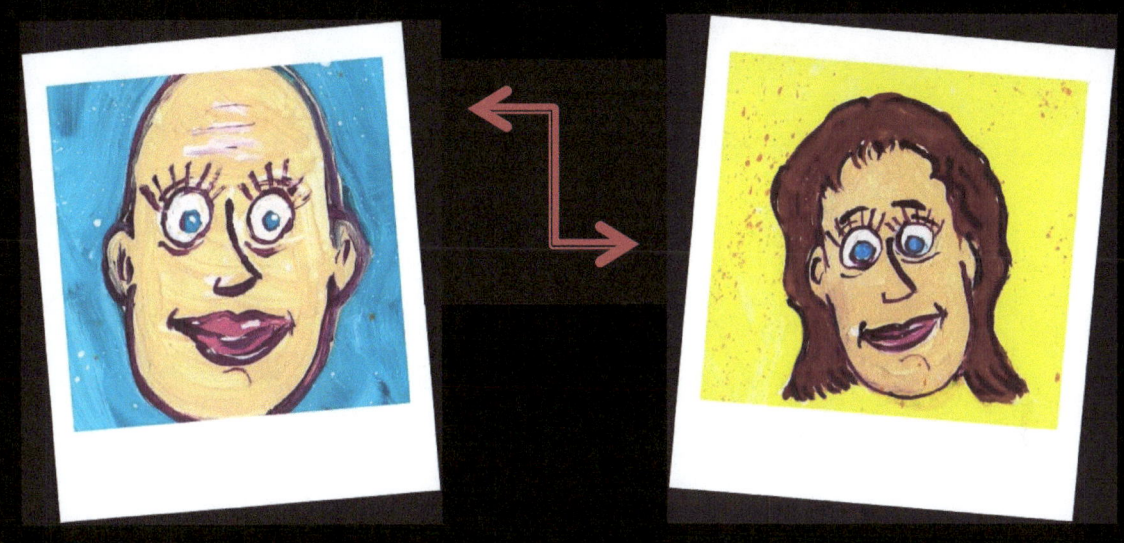

This is because chemotherapy kills cells that grow fast. Since our hair grows fast, the chemotherapy kills it too. But don't worry, their hair will grow back!

Radiation is another form of treatment that is used to treat cancer.

There are different forms of radiation.

This treatment uses high energy radiation beams to shrink tumors and kill cancer cells by damaging their

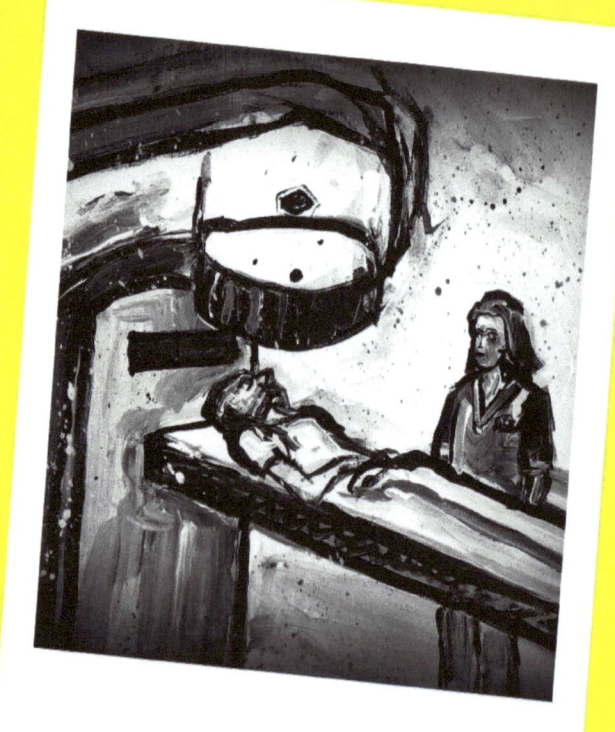

Although chemo and radiation are the most common forms of treatment for cancer, there are also others ways that people can help treat and prevent cancer.

Such as...

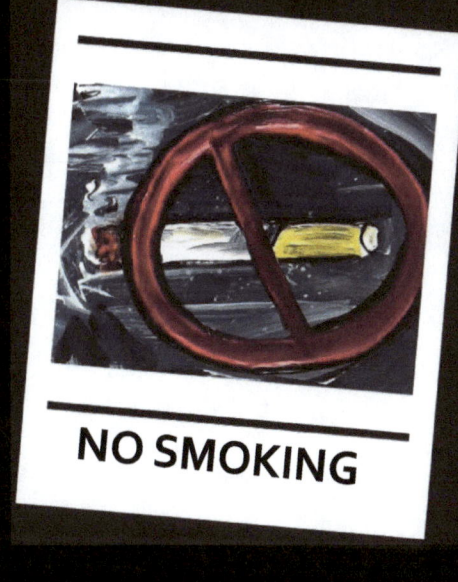

NO SMOKING

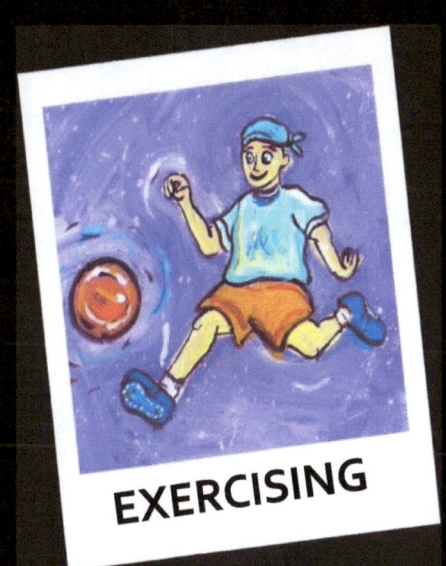

EXERCISING

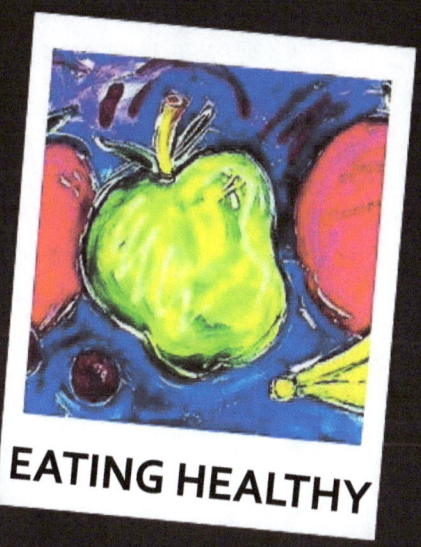

EATING HEALTHY

What Cancer **CAN** Do

- Make a cancer patient feel sick or grumpy or tired

- Cause a person to have to stay in the hospital

- Make a student miss school

- Change someone's appearance and make them look a little different

Knowing someone with cancer can cause many different feelings. These feelings can be overwhelming, especially if the person with cancer is someone in your family or a close friend.

It is okay to feel angry, sad, afraid or any of the other feelings that you may have.

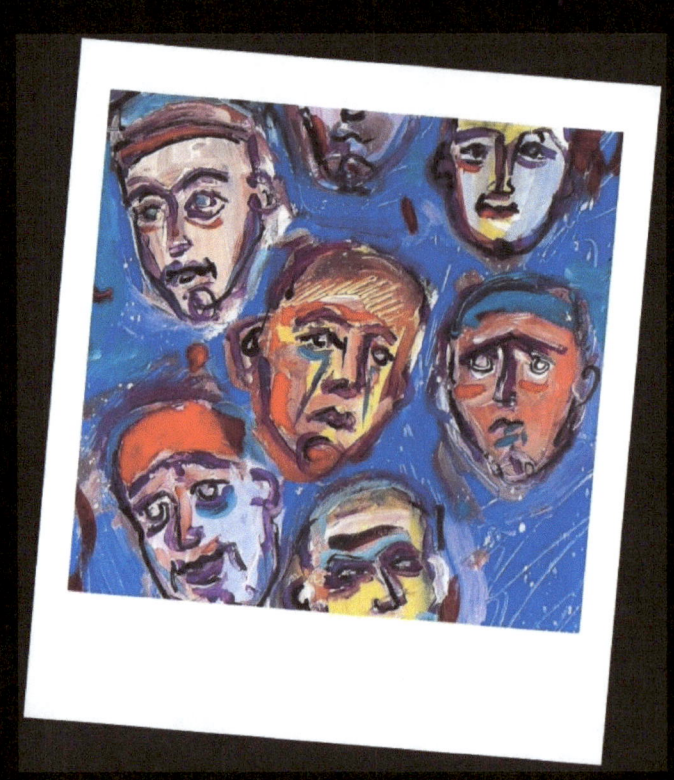

IT IS IMPORTANT THAT YOU DO NOT TREAT A PERSON ANY DIFFERENTLY THAN YOU DID BEFORE, BECAUSE THEY HAVE CANCER!

What Cancer Cannot Do

- It cannot break up friendships

- It cannot get rid of hope

- It cannot take away true beauty

- It is NOT contagious

REMEMBER –
cancer is nobody's fault!

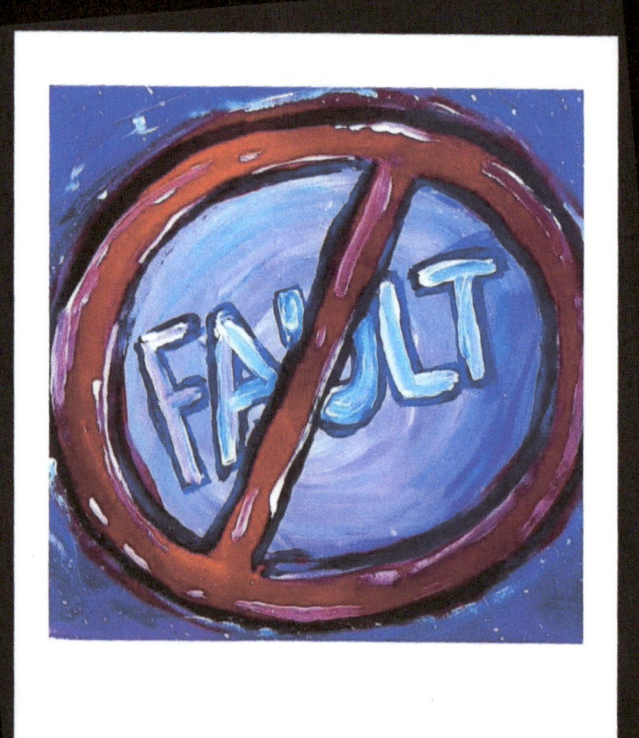

It is okay to ask questions!

If you need to talk about it, talk to your parents, your teachers or your School Counselor.

How You Can Help

Show your support by making cards or writing letters to cancer patients so that they know that you care.

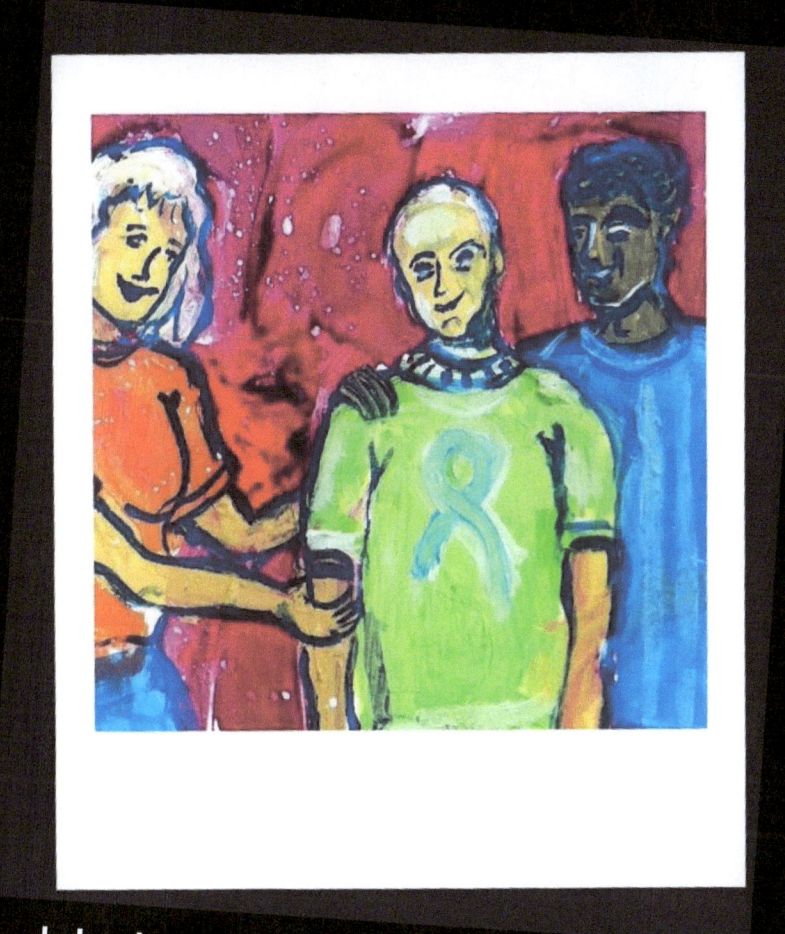

You could also do something special for the patient and their family on a holiday or on their birthday.

When able, visit the person and keep them company so that they know they are not alone.

Enlist the help of your family, friends and neighbors to collect money for someone you know who has cancer or donate it to a local

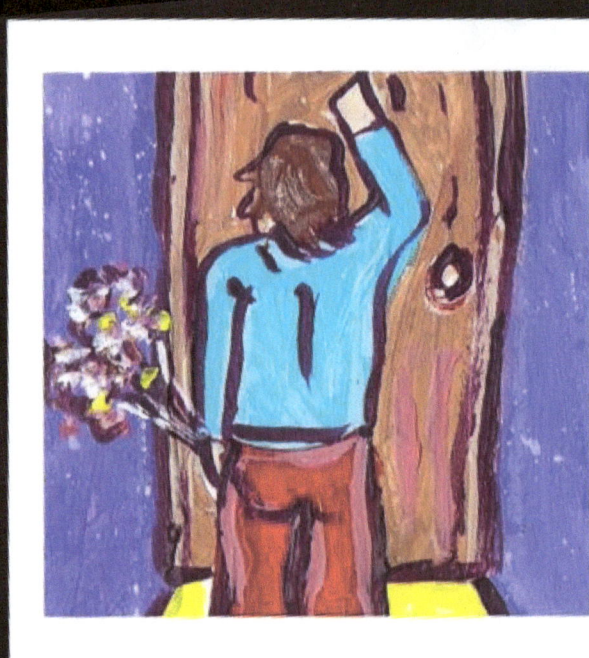

Sometimes you may feel helpless because it seems as though you cannot make the person with cancer feel better. However, just by letting that person know you are there and that you care - you are helping.

DO NOT stop reaching out and being available to them.

Cancer Awareness and Resiliency Education (C.A.R.E.)

This book is a part of a program created by Cancer Connection of Northwest Ohio, Inc. for the purpose of raising awareness and promoting resiliency in children.

The C.A.R.E. Program contains tools for personal contribution, a trait of resiliency, that allow children who may be experiencing the hardship of cancer, the opportunity to participate in a meaningful way to reach out to others.

C.A.R.E. Kits enable children to make a card, collect money, visit a cancer patient and reach out to others without fear of the disease itself.

C.A.R.E. Kits offer "positive, meaningful participation" by giving a gift of care to a loved one or to a community member with cancer!

To learn more about our C.A.R.E. Program visit our website at
www.CancerConnectionOfNorthwestOhio.com

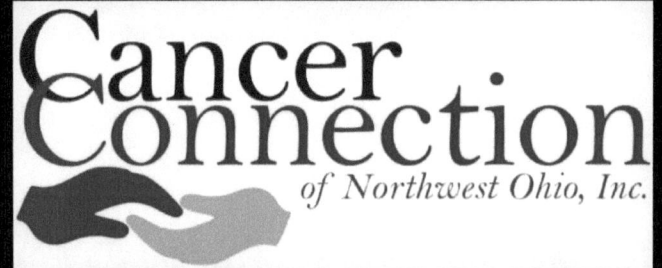

We are a 501(c)(3) non-profit organization that was created because of a personal cancer experience. Having realized a need in the community for additional support on behalf of cancer patients and families, this organization was founded in December of 2008. We are comprised of Volunteers and Board Members who are passionate about assisting others in our community.

The mission of Cancer Connection of Northwest Ohio, Inc. is to journey hand-in-hand with those who are afflicted with cancer by connecting individuals and their families to vital resources, providing hands-on support, and creating programs that meet the physical, emotional, and spiritual needs of cancer patients and their families in our community. We serve ALL cancers and ALL ages.

At Cancer Connection of Northwest Ohio, Inc., we believe it is important to take care of the whole person. We envision cancer patients and their families receiving readily available support and resources that go beyond fighting the disease itself; aid that focuses on taking care of the hearts and minds of those individuals impacted by cancer.

Our long term goal is to take this concept to other cities and assist in the creation of similar organizations that will fill the needs of those communities.

For more information or to start a Cancer Connection in your area, please visit our website at www.CancerConnectionOfNorthwestOhio.com or call us at 419-725-1100.

FROM THE ILLUSTRATOR

Unfortunately these days we all are getting too much experience with cancer. Whether it's personally or with a loved one, it seems to be all around us. As one of seven children, my first experience was when I was in my teens and my oldest brother David, who was in his early twenties and in the Navy at the time, was diagnosed with testicular cancer. He went through many surgeries, chemo, the works. Finally it got to the point where the doctors gave him 4 months to live due to the progression of his illness. I am happy to say though, due to a spiritual experience and healing, my oldest brother turned 50 this July, celebrating this with his 2-kids which he wasn't supposed to be able to have.

A few years ago however, I watched David and his wife work through his step-son Gabriel, who was age 7 at the time, be diagnosed with an extremely rare and terminal form of lung cancer. Gabe made the news, got a lot of community support, got to do a Make-A-Wish trip, and got his wings surrounded by those who love him.

My oldest sister Michelle is still working through her diagnosis of another rare form of cancer named Dermatofibrosarcoma Protuberans. Even with very visible facial scars, she's doing great with an amazing and inspiring positive attitude toward things. My younger brother Joe had that same form of skin cancer a few years back, but also had the area removed.

Knowing what my family has gone through, I understand what other families are going through when battling cancer. Over the past years, I've used my artistic gifts for fundraisers and to support fantastic organizations like Cancer Connection of Northwest Ohio. The support, education and services they provide truly are priceless. I was honored to be involved in this book project and can only encourage families going through cancer experiences to use these great resources available to them.

Greg Justus
Modern Impressionism
www.artofjustus.com

FROM THE CONTRIBUTOR

I have fond memories of my grandmother who always had a way of making me feel loved and special to her. I remember the way she would hold my hand and caress my fingers gently and say, "Don't forget how much I love you." Her favorite flower was Forget-Me-Nots and her motto in life was to "always find a way to laugh no matter what." I spent many weekends with my grandmother making up games, writing poems, telling stories and laughing.

When I was ten years old, my parents told me that my grandmother "Nanny" had cancer, to pray for her and that I could not see her until she gets better. My grandmother's cancer had spread rapidly shortly after she was diagnosed. She grew ill very quickly having extensive chemo-therapy and my parents decided it was best for me to not see my grandmother in this condition. I remember waiting in the hospital waiting rooms while my parents had short visits with her. During that time, my teacher had the whole class make get-well cards for my grandmother. I remember waiting in the car when my mom went in to take the cards to her, wanting so badly to run in the house to see her and wishing and praying. I never got a chance to see her again. My grandmother died from cancer at 49 years old. As a child, I felt a sense of guilt that maybe I did not pray enough and wondered if it was my fault.

Some years later, I met Jean Schoen of Cancer Connection of Northwest Ohio when one of my own students asked if we could do something for people with cancer. This sparked the beginning of our partnership as my own classroom students began making cards for cancer patients in the community and Jean delivered them to area hospitals during the holiday season. Since that time, we have been working together to provide children the opportunity to reach out to cancer patients and to create educational programs and cancer awareness projects to support and help teachers, parents and children. I am so honored and appreciative of the opportunity to contribute to a book for children who know someone with cancer . I am so blessed to have such a wonderful way to express the fact that indeed, I did not forget her. I hope this book holds the hand of each little one it reaches.

Julie Greenberg, M.Ed
Educator and Intervention Specialist, Oregon City Schools
President, Toledo Council of the International Reading Association

"A well written book that touches on the many issues that children face with loved ones who have cancer. An easy-to-understand book that answers many questions that children of all ages may have. Talking with children about such heavy issues can be difficult and this book helps to make it understandable for them."

Jenny Henkle, RN, BS, Oncology Nurse, Palliative Care Coordinator

"I recommend this book as an excellent resource for parents or caregivers to begin to explain cancer to children."

Julie Kujawa, M.Ed, Mother, Elementary School Teacher, Cancer Survivor

"I thought the book was very unique and thorough. Unfortunately there are limited resources that educate young children and their families, which makes this a much needed resource."

Karen Andres, Cancer Center Social Worker

"I would highly recommend Cancer Connection of Northwest Ohio, Inc. and the C.A.R.E. Program that they have created. I have found the program to be professionally done and a useful tool for explaining cancer to children of any age. As a School Counselor, I feel that this program would be valuable for others in my field. I endorse this program and feel it is a great fit into our curriculum."

Debbie Miller-Pultz, School Counselor